Herniated Discs
What Works
What Doesn't

A case study of spinal injuries, multiple herniated discs and treatments

NEERAJ MALHOTRA

Copyright © 2017-18 Neeraj Malhotra

All rights reserved.

ISBN: 1981437444
ISBN-13: 978-1981437443

DEDICATION

This book is dedicated to my mom – Promila Malhotra
Rest in peace mom, love you always.

CONTENTS

	Foreword	i
1	The Accident How it all started	3
2	The Spine Story begins here	10
3	Steroids Consume as there's no tomorrow	16
4	Injections To the point but temporary	21
5	Chiropractor Healing Touch	27
6	Toshi Making it better	33
	Epilogue	38
	About the author	39

FOREWORD

The thing that sets Neeraj apart most, is his ability to think differently from others and have some sort of second level thinking where he can visualize anything including his first level thoughts as a second person and generate quite useful insights about it. He is incredibly intelligent and you can see witty spark in his eyes. He is a keen reader of books and loves to share his learnings with others.

Probably his trait - "loves to share his learnings" that I mentioned about him above is the reason for him to write this book. There are many key lessons which he has shared in quite a detail in this book. While reading this book, a reader will get insights into the author's mindset while he was suffering severe back pains. It's truly amazing to see someone staying so focused on his goals in life even though been under intense pain for so long. He has never compromised on his duties as a son, husband, and father or as a friend. I think at his core, Neeraj believes that excelling at your task at hand, is of prime importance which will eventually be compounded to greater results in future. This is his quality which truly sets him apart from others.

Infinite thanks to Neeraj for allowing me to write this foreword and for his sincere efforts in getting this book out there for others who could learn from his experiences and save years of trouble in fighting back pains.

~ Khyati Malhotra ~

1. THE ACCIDENT

How It All Started

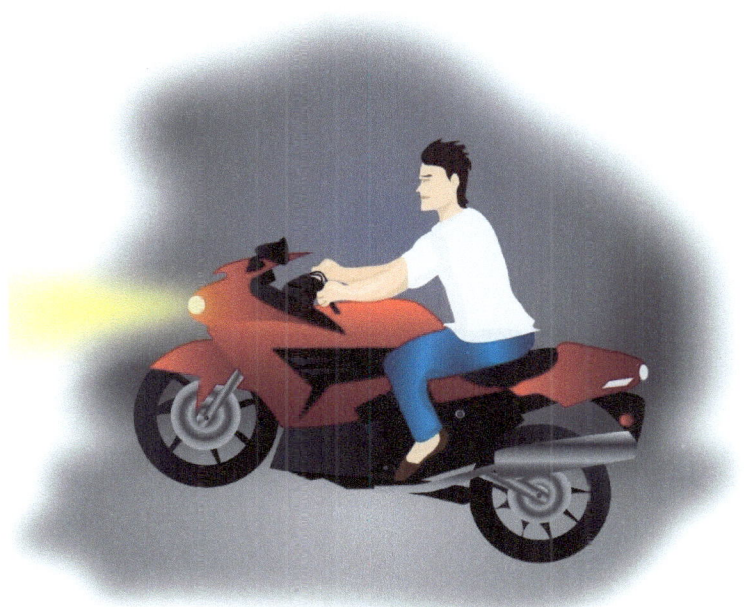

It was a Tuesday evening on 10th October 2007. After finishing a workload at office, I decided to leave for home and relax. As I was packing my stuff and ready to leave, Omkar who was working with me at same office asked me if I had any plans after work and showed his interest in joining me for the dinner. I had borrowed motor bike for the day from my other friend – Amit whom I shared an accommodation near office. Omkar and I both left the office on Amit's bike. I had been living with few friends on sharing basis in Pune; a city of India, which at the time was rapidly attracting computer engineers due to new IT corporates coming up in the city at high pace. Thus the traffic conditions had got worsen in the city and since we had decided to live closer to office to avoid long commutes between home and office, it took us just 20 minutes to reach my home.

The friends whom I was sharing a 3 bedrooms apartment in Pune, were Gyan –who I think was most calm & patient of all; Lalit – true money saver and maker & Amit – health conscious & muscle builder. I had a separate room and with limited furniture in the house, I asked Omkar to pull a chair for himself. Other friends were still not home yet. We both started talking about the future of Pune city and how we can find some good business opportunities there. I remember there were various ideas ranging from improving city conditions, facilitating commuters who stuck in traffic for many hours of the day and many software applications. We were still discussing when Gyan knocked at the door. I opened the door and found my roomies and a guest with them. I knew Rohan as he was working within same team as Gyan at our office. So, now it was four of us and two guests in the house.

Since it was dinner time, our unanimous decision was to go out to nearest restaurant, have dinner and then come back home to play UNO (a playing cards game). By 8pm we all returned home from dinner. After playing UNO for next two hours, I got bored with game and suggested others to go for late night movie show. It was hard to convince anyone as it was late and everyone was tired of working all day in the office and we all had to join office again next morning. But I was adamant and finally succeeded to convince four out of five friends. Amit didn't join us for movie that night and went to his room.

Rohan, Gyan and Lalit left on two motor bikes to get the

tickets and I was coming behind with Omkar. Since our discussion of solving city problems and finding business solutions was left in middle when others came home, so we both continued the discussion while I was driving the motor bike and he was sitting behind me and talking. As I was talking while driving, I choose to drive slower than usual. On the way to movie theatre, we met all potholes on the road we could. The potholes are quite common on Indian roads and a careful driver could avoid most of them. Since I was out of form on the day, my friend joked if I was counting all the potholes in the city by going through each one of them. This made us laugh for a while and he asked me to focus on the road. Now looking back, I think that I wasn't seeing the signs of something unusual on that day, may be a warning for what would happen soon. I continued talking and kept throwing more ideas about problems and their solutions for rest of our journey while driving carelessly.

Lesson Learned
"Be alert and focus on task in hand"

It took double the time than usual to reach Movie Theater. Our friends had bought tickets and were waiting at the gate for us. The show was starting in 5 minutes, so we rushed after parking my bike. Since cleaning staff was still working on getting theater room ready for the next show, we were asked to wait outside on stairs for few more minutes. I remember that we took some pictures of ourselves posing near movie posters on the display there, as theatre was literally empty. We watched movie which ended at around 2:30am and we all were very sleepy and very tired by that time, so we got on our bikes quickly and head for homes. Omkar sat on Rohan's bike now as they were heading to their own home and Lalit joined Gyan on his bike. I was alone on my bike.

For some time we all drove our bikes in parallel as rarely we get empty roads in busy city like Pune. After driving few blocks together, I accelerated further as if my inner voice asked me to drive faster to reach home early. I still can't answer why I did it instead of enjoying driving next to my friends. In few seconds, I accelerated to maximum speed possible on the bike, leaving my other friends far behind. I love speed and had driven bikes or cars at very high pace many times in the past. The road was clear and there was no other vehicle as far as I could see at that time. In a short while, I noticed something was there in the middle of the road about 150 - 200 yards ahead of me. Soon, I realized they were few street dogs, sitting in the middle of the road. Last I had checked, I was accelerating close to 120 kilometers per hour and I had to make a decision in split of seconds on how to approach upcoming obstacle. I can imagine that the captain of the greatest ship ever Titanic, would have got much more time than what I did, when he was informed **"captain! Iceberg ahead"**.

Ahead of me were few street dogs who were sitting in the middle of the road and if I didn't do anything soon, then definitely I would hit them and that will be disastrous at that speed for me as well as for dogs. Quickly my instincts gave me two options; slow the bike or keep driving from the sides. I thought that abruptly pushing the brakes at that high speed, might trip the bike. Moreover dogs might rush towards me in attacking mode. So, I decided on second option as the safest in the situation, which was to keep driving from the sides. I thought in my head that in such a cold night these dogs won't even realize that a bike just passed by them. So, I was very confident on my decision.

Lesson Learned

"Confidence is good. Over confidence is a killer. The challenge for anyone is to acknowledge when it's latter."

On usual days, I wore a heavy leather jacket whenever going for the bike ride with required full gear such as shoes, gloves, glasses or goggles and a helmet. But on this day, I had a cotton jacket, with floaters instead of shoes and no helmet or gloves.

Lesson Learned
"Stick to a process. Sounds boring but it can save you someday"

As I was approaching near those dogs very fast, one of them got up and started moving from the middle of the road towards the pavement on right side of the road. This was the side I had chosen to pass by. It was thin black dog and I could see it clearly under street light by now. I was so close to it and there was no time to press the breaks or change the lane. At that split second, I felt as if time had slowed and I could feel milliseconds as if they were minutes. It was too late for doing anything and the dog was right in front of me. I remember me turning bike to avoid hitting the dog but instead hitting the pavement with bike's front wheel which was an impact as if I had hit the wall head on. The rear wheel lifted from the ground in air, tripping and leading to many 360 degree rollers on the road. I had lost the grip when torque from rear wheel pushed me in air. I clearly remember rolling on bitumen road several times before coming to halt. Each time my skin was touching the road, I could feel it's been peeled off. My head itself hit the ground several times and I could barely cover it with my hands to protect it for any severe damages.

I was half conscious and shaking when my friends lifted me from middle of the road and put me on its side. I couldn't feel my legs or hands much and thought as if I was already dead. One of my friends put a piece of cloth on my head near my right eye to stop bleeding. I vaguely remember Gyan lifting and putting me on his bike with Omkar holding me from back. They made me sat on their bike in middle of themselves and took me to nearest hospital. Rohan & Lalit took accidental bike and somehow managed to drive it home.

I had injuries all over my body and hospital staff took me to the room. At hospital they first gave me some water to drink. Slowly I was recovering from unconsciousness and realized that it was a government hospital whose building looked as if it would collapse any moment. Soon a nurse came and asked me if I could hear her. She did basic checks to judge my consciousness such as counting fingers, looking left and right, etc. My eyes were swollen and I had blur vision due to blood in it. I asked nurse to clean my eyes so I could see clearly, which she did. After a while, I recovered to be more conscious and realized that nurse's hands were shaking while cleaning my wounds. I asked her how long has she been working there. To which, she mentioned it was her first week on the job. I asked her to call the doctor. She politely replied that "doctor sir had already left for the day and there's no doctor on duty in the night". This wasn't new in India to hear that someone had run away from his duties especially in a critical job such as a doctor.

Lesson Learned
"Understand what profession you are in. Switch to something else if you prefer comfort over your duties. Atleast your conscience will be clear."

Shortly, the nurse mentioned that near my right eye, there's a deep cut which would need stitches to stop bleeding. I wasn't fully confident on her shaky hands for giving me stitches. So, I told her "No. I don't want stitches. Please just put tight bandages on it". After much push back, she agreed to clean my wounds, put bandage on them and give me some pain killers to pass the night until next morning when I could visit my regular doctor. It wasn't looking much worse to me at that moment considering many injuries I had got throughout my childhood for being a very adventurous kid in past. I had few bruises on face, deep cut near right eye, bruises on hands, elbows, knees, legs and difficulty in moving hands and shoulders. We left the hospital for home, in same way as I was taken to it, sitting in middle of Omkar and Gyan on a bike.

We reached home and my friends carefully put me on the bed, asking if I wanted one of them to sleep with me in the room for the night. With strong will, I said "no I am fine! Let's go and see our regular doctor in the morning."
By the morning, the pain had worsened and all my roommates took off from office and rushed me to nearest clinic. There I got some x-rays and stitches done. Doctor had found stone granules inside deep cut near my right eye and left feet. When x-ray reports came later in the day, I had both shoulders displaced, hair line fracture in both elbows and a disc displacement in lower spine.

Lesson Learned
"Never judge a letter by its cover."

2. THE SPINE

The Story begins here

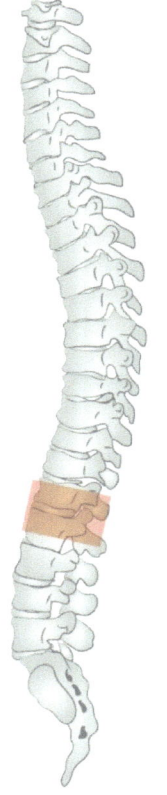

In medical terms, the spine is described as

" a series of vertebrae extending from the skull to the lower back, enclosing the spinal cord and providing support for the thorax and abdomen".

The spine is made of 33 individual bones stacked one on top of the other. Each individual bone, also known as a disc, is covered with ligaments and muscles that connect discs together and keep them aligned. The spinal column provides the main support for our body, allowing us to stand upright, bend, and twist. Protected deep inside the bones is the spinal cord which connects our body to the brain, allowing sensory signals to travel from brain to other parts of the body and facilitate various actions such movement of your arms, legs or even fingers in the hands or feet. Strong muscles and bones, flexible tendons and ligaments, and sensitive nerves contribute to a healthy spine. Keeping your spine healthy is vital if you want to live an active life without back pains. In a nonsense act of speeding and unsafe driving, I had injured one of the most vital components of my body – The Spine.

There's another important thing I learned about human brain after my super bike accident. Although human brain is a very complex system and asserts the processing capabilities equal to millions of computers put together, it behaves as an amateur when dealing with the pains. Let me explain what I meant here. God forbids but let say you got multiple injuries in your body at the same time, may be from an accident, your brain would get signals from all the injuries together as if different electrical wires are sending current to a central unit, but it will focus most on the signal which is the strongest. In other words, if your arm and leg both are injured and leg has bigger injury than the arm, then although your brain would get signals from arm and leg but it will process signal from leg first which is stronger and override pain in the arm to some extent. This sounds a little weird but it's true and can only be understood by a person going through multiple injuries at a time. It doesn't need to be as severe as broken bones; even paper cuts in multiple fingers will force brain to focus on one cut more than all others.

The reason why I mentioned this strange phenomenon of our brain is because when I had the motor bike accident I experienced exactly this way myself. Although I wasn't aware of it at that time, my injuries from broken elbow bones and stitches on the face were much more intense than shoulder or spine displacements. In fact, I didn't feel much pain in spine for couple of months which was later found to be as the most severe injury I had got during the accident.

Over next few months of treatment, my bruises were

gone, fractures in elbow were not hurting anymore and shoulders were on place. But a pain in lower back sticks around. It started with my lower back getting stiffer after few hours of stress only. It was something new which I had never experienced before. There was no reason for me to connect it with the accident as many months had already passed by the time I discovered it.

Lesson Learned
"You can only make sense of present by connecting dots in past."

I consulted various doctors in India and they all assured that there's nothing serious and probably it was due to work stress I was going through at the time. Indian doctors whom I visited assured me that there's nothing to worry about and advised me to take some rest whenever needed. I don't blame them or anyone for it. The matter of the fact is that I was stressing my back due to work pressure. Here's another important discovery I did during those times, which is this; if you are working for an employer, and you take few days off, either for sickness or marriage in the family, although they are supportive, but eventually you will end up with working late hours tomorrow. I believe the idea is to have employee cover up for the loss of time due to his absence. I have found it to be true for over 14+ years of working with corporates across globe.

Honestly, I wasn't paying much attention to my back pain as well then due to its mild and non regular nature. Once in a month, I may have to take off from work due to a sudden back pain occurred from a stressed previous day or because I lifted something heavy or just over an uncomfortable night's sleep. This continued for few months. During these times, I carelessly used some home remedies as suggested by friends and families in addition to few over the counter medicines for temporary cure. I also tried some un-coached exercises to strengthen my spine, which didn't work either.

Lesson Learned
"Health first. No Exceptions"

In meantime, due to work requirements, I relocated to Chicago, USA which is famous for its wide culture and merciless winters. I think it's normal to have some initial work pressure at new job which I definitely expected but what I didn't expect was impact of stressful work with severe winters. Chicago is also called windy city for obvious reason. It has high wind speed almost throughout the year due to its geographical position near giant Michigan Lake. While you enjoy high winds during Chicago's summers to beat the heat, but in winters the situation is totally opposite. Trust me; you don't want to spend five minutes outside during ice cold winds.

The stressful work and severe winters in new city worked together as catalyst to worsen my back pain situation. Now instead of once in a month it was once in every two weeks or so; and the only way to get relief from pain was to apply a heating pad or hot shower. Over next few months, although I realized quite late but heating pad had became a crucial part of my daily life. I had permanently affixed an electric heating pad in my chair at home and another one at my office. Every day when I went to work, I used to turn on electric heating pad whenever needed to, to get some relief from back pain. Many of my colleagues asked me to consult a doctor but I didn't feel the need as heating pads were doing their job just fine.

Lesson Learned
"Temporary solutions don't last long."

After my accident, I had been prescribed few muscle relaxers which were quite strong and could be taken in course of back pains or similar muscle pains. From time to time, I had been taking those muscle relaxers as and when back pain was unbearable. These pills were quite good, atleast they did the job what they were composed to do. Within few minutes of taking a tablet, the pain was gone atleast for next 24 hours or so. So, those pills were my life savers in case of emergency. When I searched around in Chicago, I couldn't find them available in pharmacies. So, I ordered some from India. By now, I had completely switched to regular use of heating pads and occasional use of muscle relaxers.

Lesson Learned
"Over use of anything, doesn't work in our favor"

This carried on for next few months until one day when I was sitting next to a basketball court watching my colleagues play the game. They invited me to join one of the team and play with them, which I denied considering my usual back pain situation. Even though at that moment I didn't have any back pain, but I didn't want to stress it.

After a while, I decided to head back to home, but then I thought to myself why not play one game before leaving, as I had felt bad for denying their proposal to join their game earlier. So, I joined my colleagues for a basket ball match. New teams were decided and the match was on. My team was losing by one point and when last few minutes were remaining before the buzzer sounds, I got a chance to take the shot. As I positioned myself for the shot and jumped in air towards the basket, a player from competing team rushed to stop me but instead he pushed me from my waistline while I was still in air, which caused me to fell on the concrete floor, losing our game and impacting my neck on the floor. After a while, I woke up in an emergency room at a nearby hospital.

I was literally screaming with pain for which doctor had to

give me double dose of some strong pain killers to calm me down. They ran few X-rays of my neck area and found that I had injured my neck with herniated discs in Cervical C3 section which means a spinal disc was pushed out, probably due to impact during basketball game, which is now bulging out of the spine column and pinching nearby nerves and causing severe stabbing pains. I would define this experience as say someone is hammering a nail in my spine while I am watching it.

After few days, an MRI scan followed by X-Rays was done for my lower back as well. The results of those reports showed two more herniated discs in lumber area (lower back area near tail bone). This worried me because now out of 33 spinal discs, I had 3 discs bulging out of the spinal column and pinching nerves on their sides causing severe pains. I kept thinking why all of a sudden I had three herniated discs in my spine and so I asked the doctor at the hospital. After listening to my recent history of accident, what he told me was that I might had displaced the discs earlier during the accident itself but they were not displaced or bulged enough to become this much serious. Now after basket ball accident, these discs were pushed and displaced further, enough to put pressure on side nerves causing immense pain, even more than a fracture itself.

Lesson Learned
"Know yourself – spiritually and physically".

3. STEROIDS

Consume As There's No Tomorrow

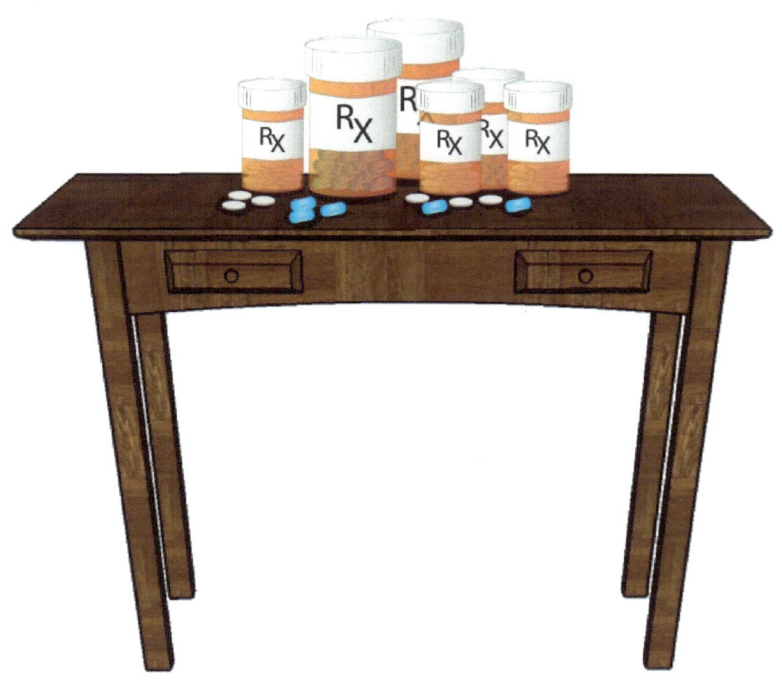

After suffering with lower back pain for almost a year and half, I had injured my spine again and this time nears my neck. As per x-ray reports, one of my cervical disc near my neck and shoulder, was displaced out of spinal column and bulged on its side nerves. As if two herniated discs in lower back were not enough and I needed one more.

At this point, it had got serious enough to get my full attention now. I realized that it's not going to heal on its own and certainly not by heating pads or ointments. So, I decided to go to the root of it and educate myself about my medical condition. So, I visited various online websites to learn about human body specifically spine and its components. Here's a quick snippet of what I think, best describes the human spine and nervous system:

Human spine is an amalgamation of vertebral column of discs and a nervous spinal cord running through it. The spinal cord is the most vital link between human brain and rest of the body. The spinal cord has two consecutive rows of nerve roots emerging on each of its sides. These nerve roots join distally to form 31 pairs of spinal nerves. The spinal cord is uniformly organized and is divided into four regions: cervical (C), thoracic (T), lumber (L) and sacral (S), each of which is composed of several segments.

The spinal nerve contains motor and sensory nerve fibers to and from all parts of the body to send and receive electrical signals. The sensory information between body parts and brain are first processed by spinal nerves. Based on the signal, the motor neurons are triggered resulting in required motion of body parts. In between the solid discs, there's a flexible jelly like material providing some cushioning. Imagine it as water filled balloon avoiding solid discs to rub against each other. When there's an uneven pressure from discs, the balloon is squeezed abnormally which causes it to bulge like a balloon is when squeezed from a side. The bulging when touches side nerves; it hinders sensory signals and causes immense pinching pain. The pain will move to other parts of the body depending upon which nerves are affected.

This was the first time; I had made an attempt to learn about my condition. Now everything that was happening with me and why it was, all of it started making lot of sense. If you are also suffering from herniated discs then above paragraph will make help you connect the dots and understand the problem a bit clearly.

Lesson Learned
"Do your own research. It will open up your mind"

When I understood that spinal cord is responsible for sending and receiving sensory signal to and from brain, it worried me to my spine. For the first time I rolled up my sleeves and decided to take proper help in fixing my spine for once and all. I immediately looked for a specialist in my area and booked an appointment. I called up my health insurance to assure that they would be covering the expenses. Health insurance provider directed me to first visit a regular physician and only if recommended to a specialist, I could proceed. What an irony that after all the premiums we pay throughout years to insurance providers, we are played like this. Even after hard attempts to convince insurer that there's lot of time already wasted, they stayed stuck on it. Anyways, I cancelled the appointment with specialist next day and made an appointment with my primary physician. Eventually, when I visited my physician, she looked up my case and understood the situation. She referred me to a specialist.

Following week, with high hopes I visited an Orthopedic as referred by physician's office. After reviewing my case and reports, he prescribed me some powerful anti-inflammatory drugs which I later found to be steroids. He explained me that those pills would resolve my issues. The results started showing up only after few days. On a scale of 0 to 10, where 0 means no pain and 10 indicates unbearable pain, my pain levels were reduced from say 9 to 5 levels which was great considering I could free my mind and focus on some other things now.

The pain was going down and so was my energy levels, I felt more sleepy and heavy head as long as I was on those medications. I researched and found some astonishing side effects of those medications and immediately stopped taking them. As they say, those side effects are just to caution patients and very small percentage of people would ever be affected.

Tip
"Those who get affected, also never imagined themselves to be part of the small percentage — that's called theory of randomness"

I had been taking muscle relaxers in the past and had understood by now that they are not going to solve the problem but rather delay it. That's why I had not liked it when orthopedic prescribed me that but he assured me that those are different and in most cases people do not need to move to next level. The way these pain killers work is simple. They slow blood flow to brain, tricking it to believe that everything is fine. This gives nature it's time to heal the body on its own. There are many people, especially doctors who won't agree with this, but that's the basic principle of pain killers.

It was already over one month since I was taking those medicines and now my pain levels had come back to 9 or even 10 on some days causing unbearable pains after I stopped taking them. It was very frustrating I looked for another doctor in my city and asked my primary physician to refer me to the new specialist. The irony was even the new specialist put me on another set of drugs and since I mentioned him already that I had been prescribed steroids in the past and they didn't help at all, he proudly said, you might not need them anymore if you take my prescribed medication for two week and in most cases, people get relief even sooner and get rid of herniated disc pains for rest of their lives.

I thought to myself that maybe it's the end of my suffering and finally I found the perfect doctor this time, I did some research about new drugs which he had prescribed me. Atleast they were not steroids which helped me gain some confidence in the specialist now. So, I continued taking those pills for next two weeks as prescribed but the results were not satisfactory.

He suggested for a refill and asked me to take same tablets for another two weeks. This continued for next three months during which he repeatedly prescribed refills of same tablets. After a month of taking steroids and three months of non-steroidal drugs, there was no cure done on core issue at all. Disappointed with their practice, I called doctor's office and expressed my disappointment and told them to stop playing with people's health. I was annoyed and in lot of pain!!

By now my back and neck pains had worsen and instead of occurring once in two weeks like before, it was constant throughout the day. Moreover, now my right arm and right leg had started staying numb for most of the time indicating that herniated discs were pushing on sensory nerves going to my right arm and leg. Numbness is really irritating especially in night as it didn't let person sleep. For temporary reliefs, I switched back to pain killers which I had bought off the counter, few sports fast relief ointment sprays and heating pad.

Lesson Learned
"Pain management is a big business in USA, which is rightly called as; 'management', not 'treatment' "

4. INJECTIONS

TO THE POINT BUT TEMPORARY

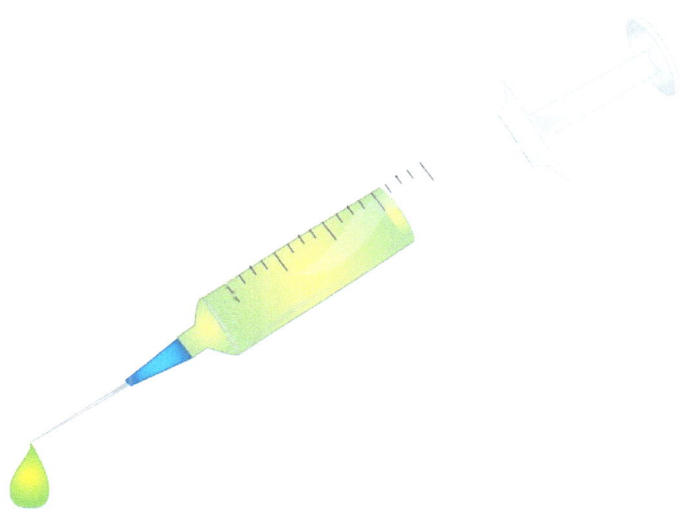

After few months I moved to Dallas due to work. Initially I missed Chicago city a lot due to its amazingly beautiful downtown and great night life. Dallas city looks quiet old in comparison to Chicago and doesn't have that great downtown and night life either. It is very different from Chicago; in terms of its culture and weather too. Initial days were quiet depressing but over next few weeks, I realized that my back pains had subdued to some lower levels without any excessive intake of pain killers or use of heating pads.

From my experience in past, I knew that muscle or fracture injuries get worsen in cold weathers, windy days and whenever there's high humidity in the air like during heavy rains. The weather in Dallas is much warmer than Chicago but fluctuates frequently. I believe the warm weather in Dallas played a major role in reducing my pain levels. This gave me hope that I may survive in this city with less or no pain killers or heat pads. Deep inside I knew that the problem with my spine hadn't been cured yet and it was just settling period which might end sometime in future.

I consider myself somewhat workaholic and as soon as I experienced better health, I started working long hours again. But unfortunately, it didn't last for long. Soon the old problems started to surface and got even more serious at this time. I had been hit much harder with back pains now. It was getting literally impossible for me to walk or stand for more than twenty minutes in a stretch. Due to lack of motion and exercise, my body weight started to increase which ultimately put more pressure on my back resulting in higher pain levels eventually. This was same nightmare which I was afraid of and had barely lived few days without it but I couldn't escape it.

Tip
"Nothing lasts forever, even bad times. Don't leave hope"

Again, I consulted my primary physician and she immediately referred me to an orthopedic surgeon specialist in spinal surgeries in the city. Before setting up the appointment, I did some research and he was one of the top surgeons in the country. Even though I wasn't in favor of surgery I decided to go and meet him.

On my first visit, he misunderstood my name for a famous Canadian NBA player – Manny Malhotra. When he came in the room and didn't find Manny sitting there, he got disappointed a little and we both joked about it for a while. He explained me how he had treated severe sports injury in the past for many players. By now, I had seen various doctors in my past for my back pain problems and so far no doctor could help me resolve it even by nominal levels. With a bit of disappointment in my voice, I asked him about his plans on treating it and how soon could I start seeing positive results.

He replied - "we would start with some anti-inflammatory for couple of weeks and if no relief by then, we would switch to stronger anti-inflammatory", which I believed he was referring to steroids. He continued with saying - "even if stronger anti-inflammatory didn't work out in our favor then he would look at my case again and discuss about further options with me".
I had gone through this kind of sessions in the past as well, so I stopped him there and said "doctor although you are an orthopedic surgeon, I do not want to go under a surgery at young age". I was just 29 at the time. He assured me that he had seen many cases like mine and he strongly believed that my condition would be cured by some tablets only and there won't be any need for a surgery. So I asked him "how those anti-inflammatory are different from what I was prescribed before by previous doctors?" He said "these are better ones, more precise and effective in curing conditions like mine". So I nodded in affirmation. Before leaving his office, I told him, that I would give it a try but I certainly didn't want you to take me to an operation bed and build up a case for the surgery.

For next three weeks, I continued taking his prescribed medications. I wasn't experiencing any relief even with new drugs. In fact as long as I had those pills into my system, the pain levels were low but as the effect of pills start fading, the pain levels were shooting to unbearable levels. I called surgeon's office and they scheduled an appointment for following week. I wasn't happy with the results of so called 'better' medication. I had strongly made it clear to the doctor in my previous sitting with him, that such medications did not work for my condition and I had been taking them for many years by now. Little bit agitated on the appointment day, I told him that "either you take some direct action to resolve the problem or I go to the next door". I was in lots of pain and all these doctors were taking same routes so far. They all were trying to solve the problem with generic medicines. It was clear to me that generic prescriptions won't help my case.

So, acknowledging my agitation, he proposed me a more intense plan of action this time. He told me that in case oral medications do not work for some patients who are experiencing pains related to herniated discs then we suggest another treatment called 'Selective Nerve Root Block (SNRB)' injections. He continued explaining that these injections are considered more effective than an oral medication because they deliver medication directly to the anatomic location that is generating the pain.

Actually it's a steroid medication which is injected to deliver a powerful anti-inflammatory solution directly to the area that is the source of pain. So, in my case it will be injected on a nerve across my spine. I am not sure about you but thinking of getting an injection in middle of your spine and that too on a nerve, was quite scary when I heard it first time. I could feel the chill in my spine while he was talking about it. I asked him about the pain that will be introduced due to those injections. He convinced me that I won't feel the pain during treatment as it would be given to me after an anesthesia shot. It is important that patient stays rock steady during this treatment as doctor would need to position the needle around the nerves and no other nerve should be touched.

My daily life was severely affected due to these back and neck pains. I had been off the work many times in last month itself. It was worrying me more than ever as the world hadn't come out of great financial recession even after 3 years in 2012. I was afraid that like other people, I might be laid off. I couldn't have that happen as I had more responsibilities now. I and my wife were blessed with a baby girl last year and I was already thinking about her future. Apart from fear of losing job, my physical activities were restricted greatly and I couldn't even lift my infant daughter or help my wife with grocery bags. I was feeling very helpless seeing her doing all the work at home. I was feeling awful emotionally now. I was tired of trying and at the verse of losing my battle against an evil of back pains. I was seeing end of my life. It was the most painful period of my life till then.

What other option did I have, so I agreed to take the spinal nerve injections. I took an appointment at hospital to get admitted few hours before the treatment. On the day, I was taken to an operating room where doctor was waiting for me. After few minutes in, nurse gave me anesthesia after which I didn't remember anything. They operated on my back and gave me two shots one at the neck area and one at my lower back, right next to herniated discs. About an hour later, I regained my conscious in same room where I was waiting before the treatment started. Nurse came in and told me that I could go home and needed to take rest for the remaining day.

I couldn't feel much my right arm and leg for next 12 hours and so had to take help from my wife to walk and use restroom. As doctor had explained me earlier that the results should appear in 2-3 days after the treatment and so it did. The pain had drastically reduced to levels of 2-3 on scale of 10. I was happy; it was the first time in last several years when

I didn't have any pain in lower back or neck. I was feeling great and ready to take the world head on. Nay, I am being over dramatic here. I was certainly better health wise and was taking all the precautions as was recommended by the surgeon. But my better looking back didn't last for more than two weeks after the treatment. Slowly, old pain started building up again and soon it reached to the earlier levels of two week before. I was depressed at that moment, very depressed.

I was angry when I met the surgeon in my next appointment with him. He persuaded me to go for another set of injections. His theory was that in my case the situation had become so worse that it would need double dose of medication through selective nerve root block injections. I agreed to go for another set of shots scheduled after few weeks. The irony was, after going through two more injections one at the back and other at neck second time, the relief didn't even last for three days. This was the end of my adventure with selective nerve root block injections. I called the surgeon's office and told them I am not coming back, not because I was treated but because I wasn't. Their final response was "I need a surgery". At last my surgeon took me where I didn't want to go. He tried to persuade me that my herniated discs needed to be removed from spine and replaced with artificial discs to fix my back problems. When I asked me what could go wrong during surgery? He mentioned about damaging some nerves which could result in lifetime paralysis. It was no brainer when I heard it, and so I hung up the phone.

Lesson Learned
"A salesman will sell what he's trained to"

5. CHIROPRACTOR

HEALING TOUCH

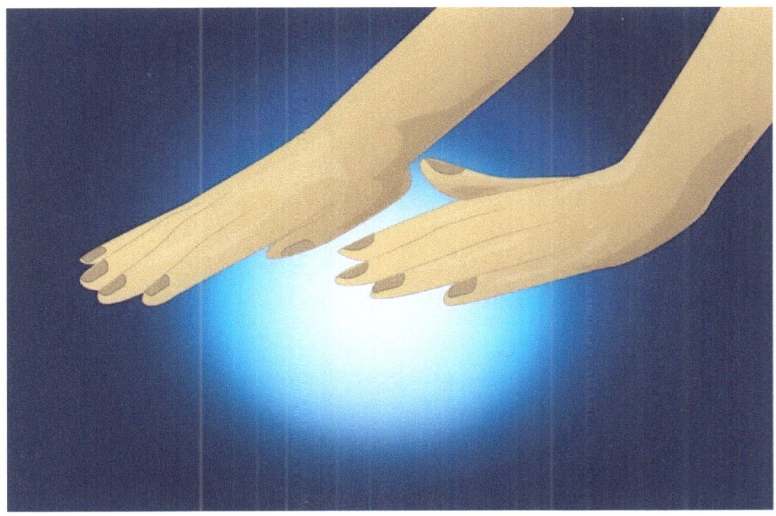

Few months had passed and I was fighting with constant back pains on daily basis. After all kinds of treatments from various specialists, I was still not able to walk ten yards without pain, or stand still at a place for five minutes. I must sit after five minutes of standing or walking. That was horrible considering I was in early thirties. It wasn't all, even lying on a bed for some time would hurt my back irrespective of my posture. This was my everyday life now. Whenever I remember those days, I realize how helpless someone can be if his body isn't functioning as expected. By now I had repented on numerous accounts of me going for the movie which was appropriately titled – "Zindagi (Life) Rocks" on that day when I had motor bike accident.

Then as if stars had shifted and on one day a miracle happened. As if God has some messenger to send me a message. Let me tell you why I referred the God for the first time in my book so far? It was a Sunday evening and I received a call from one of my brother in law who lives in Michigan. When his phone call came, I had bad back pains and was resting at home. He sensed it and asked me about how was my back doing. He asked me to send him details from my medical reports about exact problem. I think he made few phone calls right away to consult with some of his friends. Later in the night, he called me again. He told me that everyone he had checked with was suggesting me to go for a surgery, but one of the guys had advised him to see a chiropractor and inquire about the decompression therapy. I hadn't thought about going to a chiropractor before. So, I googled to find out who chiropractors are and how they can help me? This is what I found on Wikipedia about a chiropractor;

"a chiropractor is a person who practices chiropractic alternative medicine, specializing in the diagnosis, treatment and prevention of disorders of the neuro-musculoskeletal system and the effects of these disorders on general health."

So, now this was clear who a chiropractor was but I was still suspicious on how a chiropractor can fix my spinal injury? I didn't search anymore and went in different room to rest. Over the sleepless night while in pain, my brain was still trying to find answer to whether I should give chiropractor a try or just stick to my previous conclusion that nobody can treat this. In the morning, I searched internet for decompression therapy that my brother-in-law was suggesting me to find more about. I found some YouTube videos explaining how decompression therapy, also known as non-surgical spinal decompression, actually works. Basically, nonsurgical spinal decompression is a type of motorized traction that may help relieve back pain. Spinal decompression works by gently stretching the spine. That changes the force and position of the spine. This change takes pressure off the spinal disks, which are gel-like cushions between the bones in our spine, by creating negative pressure in the disc. As a result, bulging or herniated disks may retract, taking pressure off nerves and other structures in the spine. This in turn, helps promote movement of water, oxygen, and nutrient-rich fluids into the disks so they can heal.

I was astonished to find that such a treatment was possible without surgery and I didn't know about it yet. But I was still skeptical if that would be the answer to my problems. I kept researching about it for next few days as I wanted to make sure not to worsen my problem even more. My right arm and leg were already numb about 30% and that was like an add-on to suffering of lower back and neck. By now, it was clear that numbness was all related to root problem that is multiple herniated discs. So after a course of days, I discussed it with my wife and we decided to give it a shot. After assuring with my health insurance that chiropractic treatment would be covered, I looked up for best chiropractor in the area and booked an appointment.

When I reached the clinic, I requested to meet the doctor first. The staff was supportive and asked me to wait for few minutes. Soon I was shown way to doctor's office. There was a six feet plus tall man, heavy build, politely offered me a chair and asked me to explain my reason for visit. I thoroughly explained him my journey over last few years of pain and how it all started. He patiently listened and was taking notes. Before finishing, I told him that there's no way I would opt for surgery at this age unless I am about to die due to this pain. If he is also going to put me on medications and finally end up suggesting surgery then I am not interested. I believe he understood why I was a bit harsh at saying that. So he asked me for three days of time for his office to request all records from my previous visits to various doctors & clinics and to study my case. He didn't bill me for that appointment and scheduled me up for next appointment in three days.

I remember next appointment was on the day when my daughter was turning two years old. I had taken a day off to spend time with her at home. So, I took 10 am appointment at chiropractor's office. On the day of the appointment, I was sent directly to doctor's office where he explained me reason for my constant pain with pictures, disc models and drawings very clearly. I could clearly say that he had studied my case thoroughly and was speaking specific to my health problem not in general ailments and their treatments, which gave me lots of confidence in him. Unlike other doctors in the past he also mentioned that he would not be able to fix the discs 100% non-surgically but my pain levels will be drastically reduced and the pain would come to nominal levels and stay there as long as I carefully watch my activities. I liked his honesty and agreed to start the treatment.

Next he called his practitioner nurse in and instructed her to prepare me for the decompression therapy. I had studied about it in past which assured me that I was on the right path. So they took me to next room called 'kinetic room' where after some mild stretches and exercises, the nurse fits a harness belt around my pelvis and another around my trunk. With clothes on, I was asked to lie down face up on a computer controlled table. Then she hooked up the other ends of the harness to align my position as intended for the treatment. Then doctor came in to examine the harness and position of table. After that he configured some settings in a small panel controlling the table's movement, he turned it ON. For next 30 minutes, the table first extends itself to a set limit with harness belts exerting a pull on my spine and holding it in stretched position for 30 seconds and then releasing the force gently to recoup back to normal position. It wasn't painful at all but rather relieving. So I opened a book on my phone while this was going on. After 30 minutes, the computer stopped and nurse asked me to gently get up from the table. That was it!!!

After first treatment only, my pain had gone completely and I was feeling what 30 years old should. I didn't have any pain after this treatment and I thanked the doctor, scheduled next appointment as the treatment needs to be repeated for couple of weeks in order to permanently adjust the bulging disc at its normal position in the spine and left his clinic with a broad smile on my face.

When I reached home, I had a big smile on my face and my wife could tell that therapy must have relieved me from the pain. This was a rare day in my life after so many years. I was feeling very good; first it was my daughter's birthday and second, I didn't have any pain in my lower back or neck for the first time in many years. I asked my wife to get diaper bag ready for our daughter so we could go out and celebrate her birthday at some nice place. We decided to take her to a zoo which a two year would enjoy as she had started learning about animals just yet. I drove for 40 miles to the zoo and then walked about 2-3 miles inside the zoo, which wasn't possible in my wild dreams before. I was feeling as if the God had guided me to go for this treatment via my brother-in-law. I called my brother-in-law later in the day and thanked him for suggesting me to go to a chiropractor and getting decompression therapy done. I will always be thankful to him for this. I am a spiritual person myself and believe that God has wonderful ways to send us help and I believe this was one of his ways.

Lesson Learned
"Don't lose your faith in whatever you believe in"

6 TOSHI

MAKING IT BETTER

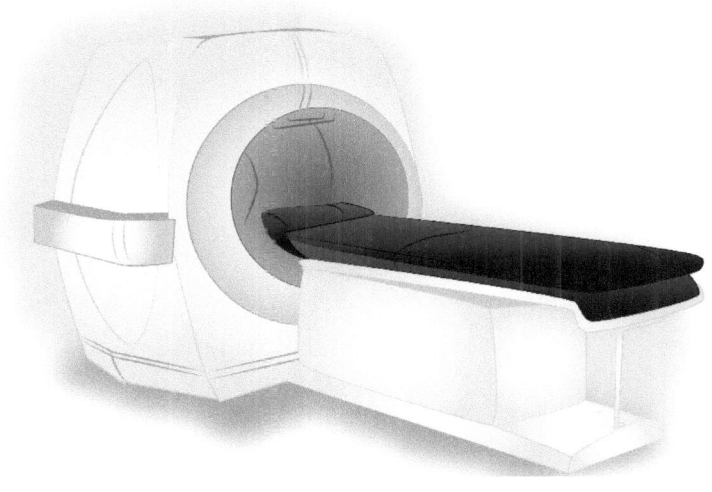

For next two years or so, I continued with decompression therapies at my chiropractor's office at Dallas. If I can remember correctly, I had over 55 and so decompression therapy sessions over this period. As I have explained that in the decompression therapy a harness belt is placed around patient's hips and is attached to the lower side of a motorized table near the feet and upper part of the table remains in a fixed position while the lower half of the table, to which the patient is harnessed, slides back and forth to provide traction and relaxation. There can be many different positions in which a patient is attached a harness and connected to the table.

After so many therapies, the pain levels had reduced from unbearable levels of 9 out of 10 to 3 out of 10 or less But the problem was that the pain hadn't gone completely. Although pains levels and frequency had reduced to comfortable levels but there were still occasions when a wrong move or posture in sleep could result in shifting of spinal discs and causing extreme pains. Remember I was told by Chiropractor that I need to watch out my activities. I also noticed that my posture had changed a bit and spine was bending more than usual.

In few days, I had to travel overseas for a wedding in family. The exertion from wedding had started showing effects on my back and as if all of sudden unbearable pains in lumber and cervical areas had come back. I was in lots of pain in middle of all family functions. Soon, my elder brother found a doctor in the city who had a good rapport from his past patients. He scheduled me an appointment with him for emergency visit next day. I expressed my concern to him that after so many decompression therapies I took in last two years, my spine should have adjusted better to avoid future displacement of the discs. New doctor was an expert in pain management and served non-surgical treatments to his patients suffering from orthopedic ailments. He patiently listened to me and asked me to bend forward as much as I could comfortably try to touch my feet. While I bent, he observed my spine and made some marks with a pen on my back. While I was still bent, he brought a tool called activator & adjustor which I had seen my chiropractor using as well on me. The Activator, a small hand held tool, is designed to deliver a gentle impulse force to the spine with the goal of restoring motion to the targeted spinal vertebra or joint. When he used this tool and gently pushed on my spine, it worked as a magic and immediately I could bend even more with no pain in the back. I imagined this tool as a magic wand given to chiropractors and pain management specialists.

I was ready to get back to family functions and take the dance floor. Doctor asked me for how many days, would I be in the city and be available for some therapies. He treated me with something called "Pulsed Signal Therapy" or commonly abbreviated as PST, over next few days. This therapy was different from chiropractor's decompression therapy. In PST, the patient is exposed to unnoticeable electrical signals. As a patient, I didn't feel any pain or electric shocks while going through this therapy. Basically, in this pulsed signal therapy, small impulses of electrical signals with specific strength, intensities and frequencies are focused on affected areas of a patient's body. Each pulse induces a tiny electrical signal that stimulates cellular repair. Based on my experience, you can take a nap while lying on the table during the therapy and it takes approximately 45-60 minutes for each session.

Although pulsed signal therapy makes uses of magnetic field for the treatment, these fields are very low frequencies and don't feel at all on the surface. I learned that PST can treat joint problems, arthrosis, rheumatism, back pains and sports injuries. He suggested me that I would need 12 sessions on consecutive days to complete the therapy. I was also warned that if the treatment is interrupted for more than 48 hours, you shall have to start from session one. That's how this therapy works and slowly helps in repairing the tissues non-surgically.

But my question remained with him that why I had so much of pain all of a sudden and why didn't tens of decompression therapies help me in making the spine stronger? He responded that as I had gone through so many decompression therapies, my spine had actually got weaker with the time. This also explained the reason for bending of my spine. It had bent to an extent that anyone could notice a forward bend in my posture even while standing or walking.

He also explained that decompression therapy is very helpful in treating herniated discs and other issues but in my case, I might have done it more than required and I must be less aggressive on it. He recommended me PST therapy to repair the cellular tissues in the lumbar spine with another treatment to correct the posture. As per him, once the posture is corrected, I would stop putting uneven pressure on few of the discs and instead balance evenly over the spine avoiding more discs to bulge out and be displaced.

I continued with sessions and results were promising. He asked me to go through these sessions at least once in a year to keep the spine in check in addition to the decompression therapy. I will visit him again next time I am in India.

I would recommend anyone who is suffering by herniated discs to research more about PST therapy and find a doctor nearby. I hope my story would encourage others to explore more options instead of surgery and never lose their hope.

Lesson Learned

"Never ever lose hope"

EPILOGUE

I am neither a medical practitioner nor am endorsing anyone. I just wanted to share with you what worked in my case and what didn't. I am also not saying that my herniated discs are cured and they are as new ones. Whether a patient prefers a surgery or opts for non-surgical treatments varies from person to person and his/her medical conditions.

The purpose of writing this book was to share my experience with you so that you can learn from it and do not have to go through countless steroids, injections and lots of pain for years and before it gets worse. Before you decide to go for surgery, you should consider all pros and cons of it. I believe my decision was right to take alternative medicines route because it helped me walked, stand, sit and sleep at night better than other treatments did. Above all, I can occasionally carry my daughter in arms and love her. On some days, my pain comes back but it happens now in weeks instead of daily constant pain in lower back and neck as was before. This allowed me function a little better and let me live my life happily.

ABOUT THE AUTHOR

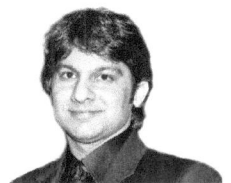

In addition to graduating with honors from a leading engineering university, Neeraj Malhotra has worked as a senior business analyst and data architect for designing and developing various challenging software solutions and products for world's giants such as AT&T, T-Mobile, Sprint and more. He grew up in India and now lives with his wife and two daughters in Texas USA. By turns, he is an engineer, prolific inventor, an author, a dad and a fledging yogi.

www.ingramcontent.com/pod-product-compliance
Lightning Source LLC
Chambersburg PA
CBHW040332220526
45473CB00009B/2655